YOUR KNOWLEDGE HAS VALUE

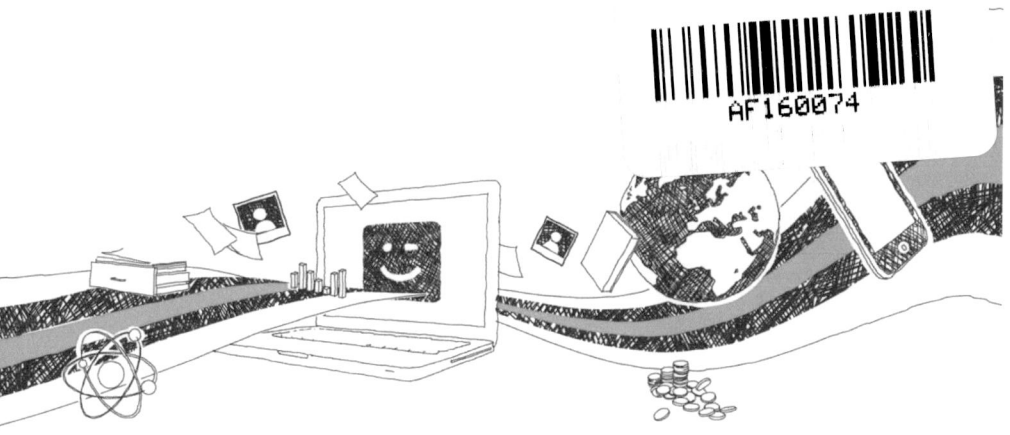

- We will publish your bachelor's and master's thesis, essays and papers

- Your own eBook and book - sold worldwide in all relevant shops

- Earn money with each sale

Upload your text at www.GRIN.com
and publish for free

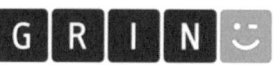

Bibliographic information published by the German National Library:

The German National Library lists this publication in the National Bibliography; detailed bibliographic data are available on the Internet at http://dnb.dnb.de .

This book is copyright material and must not be copied, reproduced, transferred, distributed, leased, licensed or publicly performed or used in any way except as specifically permitted in writing by the publishers, as allowed under the terms and conditions under which it was purchased or as strictly permitted by applicable copyright law. Any unauthorized distribution or use of this text may be a direct infringement of the author s and publisher s rights and those responsible may be liable in law accordingly.

Imprint:

Copyright © 2018 GRIN Verlag
Print and binding: Books on Demand GmbH, Norderstedt Germany
ISBN: 9783668642881

This book at GRIN:

https://www.grin.com/document/413335

Patrick Kimuyu

Alcohol Consumption and Risky Sexual Behavior amongst Adolescents and Young Adults

GRIN Verlag

GRIN - Your knowledge has value

Since its foundation in 1998, GRIN has specialized in publishing academic texts by students, college teachers and other academics as e-book and printed book. The website www.grin.com is an ideal platform for presenting term papers, final papers, scientific essays, dissertations and specialist books.

Visit us on the internet:

http://www.grin.com/

http://www.facebook.com/grincom

http://www.twitter.com/grin_com

Name: Patrick Kimuyu

ALCOHOL CONSUMPTION AND RISKY SEXUAL BEHAVIOR AMONGST

ADOLESCENTS AND YOUNG ADULTS

Introduction 2
Correlation between Alcohol Consumption and Risky Sexual Behavior amongst Adolescents
and Young Adults 2
Alcohol Consumption and Risky Sexual Behavior 3
Major Theories Explaining the Correlation between Alcohol Use and Risky Sexual Behavior
.... 4
Research Evidence 5
Consequences of Alcohol Consumption and Risky Sexual Behavior 7
Contracting sexually transmitted diseases 7
Unplanned pregnancies 8
Other health problems 9
Academic performance 9
Conclusion 10
Works Cited 11

Introduction

In retrospect, substance use and sexual activity are quite common amongst adolescents and young adults. As such, it is emerging that sexual health amongst adolescents and young adults is seemingly becoming a significance public health challenge (Cottonham 1). Owing to the high rates of risky sexual behavior and alcohol use amongst adolescents and young adults, extensive scientific inquiry has focused on investigating the consequences of these issues. Of concern has been the correlation between the co-occurrence of alcohol use and risky sexual behavior with the transmission of sexually transmitted diseases including HIV/AIDS. It is also worth noting that alcohol use has a negative influence on protection against STDs because it impairs the use of protective barriers. Given that adolescents and young adults exhibit a high tendency of sexual risk taking, alcohol use exacerbates the issue of risky sexual behaviors in these groups. Morrison et al. claim that teenagers in the US "do not consistently protect themselves from sexually transmitted diseases (STDs) or unintended pregnancy" (162). This explains the magnitude of the problem. Therefore, this paper provides a comprehensive critical analysis on the correlation between alcohol use and risky sexual behaviors amongst the young adults and adolescents. It will also discuss the consequences associated with alcohol use and risky sexual behavior amongst these groups.

Correlation between Alcohol Consumption and Risky Sexual Behavior amongst Adolescents and Young Adults

Over the past decades, alcohol use has been linked to the occurrence of risky sexual behaviors. Marrison et al. claim that alcohol use is considered as a significant factor that has led to an increased risk of HIV infection among adolescents (162).

Alcohol Consumption and Risky Sexual Behavior

Cottonham carried a systemic review of literature on the influence of alcohol consumption on risky sexual behavior amongst young adults and teenagers and found compelling evidence of positive correlation. In his review, several studies revealed that most college students tend to engage in risky sexual behavior while under the influence of alcohol. Additionally, other studies indicated that alcohol consumption amongst college students increases the risk of having unprotected sex (5). This revelation led to an extensive research on the underlying aspects related to alcohol consumption that increases the occurrence of risky sexual behaviors amongst this group. As a result, several alcohol related factors were elucidated as the driving forces behind the high rates of alcohol use and engaging in risky sexual behaviors. Cooper discusses several alcohol related factors which are considered to be responsible for the occurrence of risky sexual behaviors amongst drinkers. First, he claims that alcohol increases chances of engaging in sexual activity. In this context, alcohol is believed to create an environment that promotes sexual activity due to its physical, social and psychological aspects. Second, he claims that alcohol promotes the perception of sexual experiences. This aspect is associated to the influence of alcohol which tends to disinhibit sexual risk taking. In reality, people lose control over their consciousness while under the influence of alcohol. This implies that they become less concerned on the risks associated with their social or sexual behavior. Finally, Cooper observes that alcohol use increases the possibility of engaging in risky sexual behavior (21). In theory, these are referred to as sex related alcohol expectancies.

Major Theories Explaining the Correlation between Alcohol Use and Risky Sexual Behavior

From a theoretical approach, the relationship between alcohol use, sex related expectancies and risky sexual behavior can be explained through the use of the Alcohol Myopia Theory and the Alcohol Expectancy Theory. As discussed by Cottonham, the alcohol myopia theory holds that intoxication with alcohol creates a conflict between positive and negative outcomes. An individual who is under the influence of alcohol experiences sexual arousal and attraction as the positive outcomes. In contrast, these positive outcomes are associated with negative sexual cues such as contracting STDs and other health problems (11). It can also lead to unplanned pregnancies. In other words, alcohol favors positive sexual cues by increasing ones attention to them while masking the negative sexual cues (Lewis et al. 234). This way, the alcohol myopia theory attempts to explain the relationship between risky sexual behavior and alcohol use.

The second theory that explains the correlation between alcohol use and risky sexual behavior is the alcohol expectancy theory. As discussed by Cottonham, alcohol expectancy theory holds alcohol expectancies have a positive influence on sexual behavior. As such, alcohol increases the desire for sexual experiences. Therefore, it is presumed that individuals with strong beliefs on the positive effects of alcohol are more likely to engage in sexual behavior while under the influence of alcohol than those who exhibit weaker beliefs (Gilmore et al. 954). In this case, the alcohol expectancy theory attempts to explain how sex related alcohol expectancies promote risky sexual behavior.

Research Evidence

Owing to the significance of alcohol use and risky sexual behavior amongst young adults and adolescents, a vast literature on the topic exists that provide evidence on the correlation between the two constructs. Despite the variation in methodological approaches adopted by different researchers to investigate the relationship between alcohol use and risky sexual behavior amongst teenagers and young adults, as well as the general population, most studies show a significant relationship between the two constructs.

In one prospective study that was conducted teenage African American females in the US to investigate the correlation between substance use and risky sexual behavior, a significant correlation was confirmed. This study involved 158 participants, aged between 12 and 19 years, who were recruited from family planning and health clinics, most of whom were seeking treatment for STDs or birth control. Overall, findings of this study showed a significant correlation between substance use and risky sexual behavior, $r = .43$, $p < .01$. Similar correlation was obtained by Baskin-Sommers and Sommers who investigated the relationship between substance use and the risk of having multiple sexual partners and the likelihood of engaging in unprotected sex amongst college students. This study involved 243 participants aged between 18 and 24 years from diverse races. The results of this study indicated that students who consumed alcohol in the 6-months period were more likely to have multiple sexual partners. A significant correlation of $r = .21$, $p < .01$ between alcohol use and risky sexual behavior was confirmed, indicating that alcohol consumption influences the prevalence of STDs and HIV infection. In addition, it was found out that participants were likely to engage in unprotected sex (610).

In another cross-sectional study that was carried out by Choudhry et al. to investigate correlation between alcohol use and risky sexual behavior amongst college students, there was a significant correlation between the two constructs. This study sought to investigate the influence of alcohol use on risky sexual behavior in males and females, separately. Based on the odds ratio (OD), there was a significant correlation between alcohol use and inconsistent condom use with multiple partners. Overall, females had a high risk of inconsistent condom use while under the influence of alcohol compared to males. As such, investigators in this study elucidated two main conclusions that reaffirm the findings of previous studies which found significant correlation between alcohol use and risky sexual behavior. First, it was concluded that situational use of alcohol was significantly associated with unprotected sexual activity. Second, alcohol use was found to be related with risky sexual behavior, especially having multiple sexual partners (128).

Grossman and Markowitz investigated the effect of alcohol use on birth control and condom use among teenagers and documented a significant correlation. Overall, alcohol use was found to be associated with unsafe sex. According to the findings of this study, 50% of males who engaged in binge drinking within the past three months had sex. On the other hand, 34% of females who were involved in binge drinking were reported to have sex (390). It was also found out that teenagers of both genders who used alcohol were unlikely to use birth control and condoms during sexual intercourse compared to those who do not use alcohol and other drugs (391). In general, binge drinking was positively related to sexual activity, as well as having multiple sexual partners.

Systemic reviews have also found a significant relationship between alcohol use and risky sexual behavior in teenagers, as well as, the general public. For instance, Vagenas et al. carried out a systemic review in which they selected 30 studies from a pool of 561 articles. Of the 30 articles used for the review, 27 studies showed a positive relationship between alcohol use and risky sexual behavior. In contrast, only 3 studies showed no relationship between the two variables. However, these studies attributed this outcome to the effectiveness of public health awareness of safe sex (268-269).

Finally, Gerbi's et al. study reaffirms that alcohol use influences sexual behavior. This study presents the case in the general population, primarily amongst AIDS patients. In principle, investigators in this study aimed at identifying the relationship between alcohol consumption and two risky sexual behavior indicators: inconsistent condom use and multiple sexual partners. On the one side, alcohol use was positively correlated with inconsistent condom use ($p=< .0001$) (96). Participants who consumed alcohol were likely to engage in unprotected sex compared to abstainers. On the other side, the frequency of alcohol use was correlated with the number of sexual partners ($p= .003$). Additionally, this study showed no significant variations across races (97).

Consequences of Alcohol Consumption and Risky Sexual Behavior

From an epidemiological perspective, the co-occurrence of alcohol consumption and risky sexual behavior has devastating consequences on adolescents and young adults, as it is the same case within the general public. However, it is worth noting that each variable has its independent consequences. On the one hand, alcohol consumption is associated with risks of their kinds. On the other hand, sex related behaviors exhibit different patterns of risky behavior outcomes.

Contracting sexually transmitted diseases

One of the most devastating consequences of alcohol consumption and risky sexual behavior amongst the adolescents and young adults is contracting STDs. It is apparent that STDs are common amongst these age groups compared to the other age groups. This phenomenon is attributable to the fact that adolescents and young adults are high sex risk takers. In addition, these groups have reduced access to sexual health services, and this has emerged as a significant barrier the adolescents' health and wellbeing. In most cases, alcohol consumption amongst adolescents and young adults has been linked with increased prevalence of STDs. Diseases such as gonorrhea; syphilis, Human Papilloma Virus infection, and HIV infection have been identified as the common infections among adolescent and young adult drinkers. In a study by Hutton et al. which investigated the relationship between alcohol consumption and sexual behavior showed that gonorrhea was 5 times higher among drinkers, primarily women, compared to non-drinkers. However, men were found to have high rates of STDs and risky sexual behaviors (2012). This implies that some STDs exhibit diverse epidemiological trends amongst different groups. According to World Health Organization, alcohol use increases the vulnerability to STIs, including HIV (7). It is noted that teenager who engage in alcohol consumption tend to experiment with sexual activities. As such, adolescents and young adults are considered as high-risk groups, especially in relation to HIV vulnerability. In general, WHO observes that alcohol use combined with high rates of risk taking amongst the adolescents increases their risk of contracting HIV, as well as STIs (9). Similarly, a research by Wildsmith et al. found out that more than 1 in every 7 young adults in their study had STD (2). This aspect is attributable to several factors. First, adolescents and young adults are known to mix alcohol with sexual activities (Singh and Das 69). Second, alcohol use amongst adolescents impairs consistent use of protection such as condoms. Therefore, the high rates of inconsistent condom use increases the risk of contracting STIs and HIV/AIDS.

Unplanned pregnancies

Consequently, the co-occurrence of alcohol use and risky sexual behavior amongst young adults and adolescents leads to social problems. Of concern is the prevalence of unplanned pregnancies. In reality, teenage pregnancies have always been a significant social problem in the US, as well as other countries. As reported by Kaiser Family Foundation, over

50% of teenage pregnancies occur due to alcohol use (2). This outcome is attributable to unsafe sex amongst adolescents and young adults. In most cases, adolescents engage in sexual activities due to peer pressure. This raises the risk of carrying unplanned pregnancies due to the low level of contraceptives amongst adolescents.

Other health problems

Co-occurrence of alcohol use and risky sexual behavior is also associated with other health problems such as infertility and cervical cancer. In most cases, untreated STDs lead to devastating health consequences. For instance, untreated syphilis may cause infertility in females. On the other hand, HPV is associated with the cause of cervical cancer among females (Wildsmith et al. 1). This virus is highly prevalent among adolescents and young adults with risky sexual behaviors such as having multiple sexual partners and engaging in unprotected sex. However, it is worth noting that men act as carriers of HPV; thus females with multiple sexual partners, primarily males, increase their risk of contracting the virus, which in turn, increases their risk of developing cervical cancer.

Academic performance

Finally, co-occurrence of alcohol consumption and risky sexual behavior affects academic performance of adolescents and young adults, negatively. Over the decades, alcohol use among students has always been linked with reduced academic performance (Yörük and Yörük 3). Similarly, risky sexual behavior amongst teenagers leads to teenage pregnancies. As a result, the affected teenagers are forced to discontinue their education. For those who resume learning after the pregnancy, parenting responsibilities interfere with their education, and the ultimate outcome is poor academic performance.

Conclusion

In a brief conclusion, it is apparent that sexual health of adolescents and young adults requires exceptional attention from public health. Of concern is the increasing health costs associated with risky sexual behaviors amongst members of these groups. However, preventive approaches should focus on reducing both risky sexual behaviors and alcohol consumption. The scientific rationale for this recommendation is based on the fact that alcohol use amongst adolescents and young adults increases risky sexual behaviors. Based on systemic literature review on the correlation of alcohol use and risky sexual behavior, it is apparent that there is a significant correlation between these two variables. On the other hand, the co-occurrence of alcohol consumption and risky sexual behavior is associated with several consequences, including contracting STDs, unplanned pregnancies, infertility, cervical cancer, and reduced academic performance. Therefore, future policy interventions should focus on reducing alcohol consumption and risky sexual behaviors as interrelated variables.

Works Cited

Baskin-Sommers, Arielle and Sommers Ira. "The co-occurrence of substance use and high-risk behaviors." *Journal of Adolescent Health* 38(2006): 609-611. Print.

Choudhry, Vikas, Agardh Anette, Stafström Martin and Östergren, Per-Olof. "Patterns of alcohol consumption and risky sexual behavior: a cross-sectional study among Ugandan university students." *BMC Public Health* 14(2014):128. Print.

Cooper, Lynne. "Does drinking promote risky sexual behavior? A complex answers to a simple question." *Current Direction in Psychological Science* 15.1(2006): 19 – 23. Print.

Cottonham, Danielle 2016, "Sex-Related Alcohol Expectancies, Alcohol Consumption, and Risky Sexual Behavior among African American College Women." Master's Theses, University of Southern Mississippi 2016. *The Aquila Digital Community*. Web. 20 Nov. 2017.

Gerbi, Gemechu, Habtemariam Tsegaye, Tameru Berhanu, Nganwa David and Robnett Vinaida. "The correlation between alcohol consumption and risky sexual behaviors among people living with HIV/AIDS." *J Subst Use* 14.2(2009): 90–100. Print.

Gilmore, Amanda, George William, Nguyen Hong, Heiman Julia, Davis Kelly and Norris Jeanette. "Influences of situational factors and alcohol expectancies on sexual desire and arousal among heavy-episodic drinking women: Acute alcohol intoxication and condom availability." *Archives of Sexual Behavior* 42.6(2013): 949 – 959. Print.

Grossman, Michael and Markowitz Sara. "I Did What Last Night?! Adolescent Risky Sexual Behaviors and Substance Use." *Eastern Economic Journal* 31.3 (2005): 383-4-5. Print.

Hutton, Heidi, McCaul Mary, Santora Patricia, Erbelding Emily. "The Relationship between Recent Alcohol Use and Sexual Behaviors: Gender Differences among STD Clinic Patients." *Alcohol Clin Exp Res* 32.11(2008): 2008–2015. Print.

Kaiser Family Foundation 2002, *Substance Use and Sexual Health among Teens and Young Adults in the U.S.* PDF file. 19 Nov. 2017. < https://kaiserfamilyfoundation.files.wordpress.com/2002/01/3213.pdf>

Lewis, Melissa, Rees Michael, Logan Diane, Kaysen Elizabeth and Kilmer Jason. "Use of drinking protective behavioral strategies in association to sex-related alcohol negative consequences: The mediating role of alcohol consumption." *Psychology of Addictive Behaviors* 24.2(2010): 229 – 238. Print.

Marrison, Mary, Gillmore Rogers, Hoppe Marilyn, Gaylord Jan, Leigh Barbara and Rainey Damien. "Adolescent Drinking and Sex: Findings from a Daily Diary Study." *Perspectives on Sexual and Reproductive Health* 35.4(2003):162–168. Web. 19 Nov. 2016.

Singh Stephen and Das Arup. "Interface of Alcohol and Risky Sexual Behavior among Adolescents and Youth in Low Income Slums of Mumbai, India."*The Journal of Family Welfare* 57.2 (2011): 61-71. Print.

Vagenas, Panagiotis, Lama Javier, Ludford Kaysia, Gonzales Pedro, Sanchez Jorge and Altice Frederick. "A systematic review of alcohol use and sexual risk-taking in Latin America." *Rev Panam Salud Publica* 34.4(2013):267–74. Print.

WHO, 2005, *Alcohol Use and Sexual Risk Behavior: A Cross-Cultural Study in Eight Countries.* PDF file. 19 Nov. 2017. <http://www.who.int/substance_abuse/publications/alcohol_sexual_risk_crosscultural.pdf>

Wildsmith, Elizabeth, Schelar Erin, Peterson Kristen and Manlove Jennifer 2010, *Sexually Transmitted Diseases among Young Adults: Prevalence, Perceived Risk, and Risk-Taking Behaviors.* PDF file. 20 Nov. 2017. < http://www.childtrends.org/wp-content/uploads/2013/06/2010-10SexuallyTransmittedDisease.pdf>

Yörük, Ceren and Yörük Barıs. "Alcohol consumption and risky sexual behavior among young adults: Evidence from minimum legal drinking age laws." *Journal of Population Economics* 28.1 (201): 1–33. Print.

YOUR KNOWLEDGE HAS VALUE

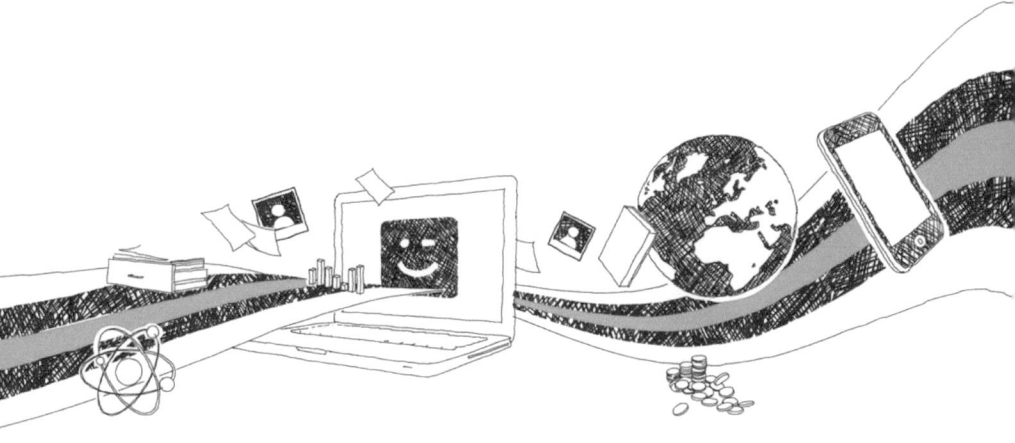

- We will publish your bachelor's and master's thesis, essays and papers

- Your own eBook and book - sold worldwide in all relevant shops

- Earn money with each sale

Upload your text at www.GRIN.com
and publish for free

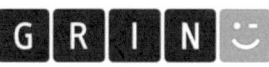